Eat 8 Hours, Fast 16 Diet

A Beginner's 14-Day Step-by-Step Guide to Intermittent 16/8 Fasting with a Meal Plan

mf

copyright © 2020 Bruce Ackerberg

All rights reserved No part of this book may be reproduced, or stored in a retrieval system, or transmitted in any form or by any means, electronic, mechanical, photocopying, recording, or otherwise, without express written permission of the publisher.

Disclaimer

By reading this disclaimer, you are accepting the terms of the disclaimer in full. If you disagree with this disclaimer, please do not read the guide.

All of the content within this guide is provided for informational and educational purposes only, and should not be accepted as independent medical or other professional advice. The author is not a doctor, physician, nurse, mental health provider, or registered nutritionist/dietician. Therefore, using and reading this guide does not establish any form of a physician-patient relationship.

Always consult with a physician or another qualified health provider with any issues or questions you might have regarding any sort of medical condition. Do not ever disregard any qualified professional medical advice or delay seeking that advice because of anything you have read in this guide. The information in this guide is not intended to be any sort of medical advice and should not be used in lieu of any medical advice by a licensed and qualified medical professional.

The information in this guide has been compiled from a variety of known sources. However, the author cannot attest to or guarantee the accuracy of each source and thus should not be held liable for any errors or omissions.

You acknowledge that the publisher of this guide will not be held liable for any loss or damage of any kind incurred as a result of this guide or the reliance on any information provided within this guide. You acknowledge and agree that you assume all risk and responsibility for any action you undertake in response to the information in this guide.

Using this guide does not guarantee any particular result (e.g., weight loss or a cure). By reading this guide, you acknowledge that there are no guarantees to any specific outcome or results you can expect.

All product names, diet plans, or names used in this guide are for identification purposes only and are the property of their respective owners. The use of these names does not imply endorsement. All other trademarks cited herein are the property of their respective owners.

Where applicable, this guide is not intended to be a substitute for the original work of this diet plan and is, at most, a supplement to the original work for this diet plan and never a direct substitute. This guide is a personal expression of the facts of that diet plan.

Where applicable, persons shown in the cover images are stock photography models and the publisher has obtained the rights to use the images through license agreements with third-party stock image companies.

Table of Contents

Introduction	7
What Is Intermittent 16/8 Fasting?	10
Principles of the Intermittent 16/8 Fasting Method	10
Benefits of the Intermittent 16/8 Fasting Method	11
Disadvantages	12
How Does the Intermittent 16/8 Fasting Work?	14
Use Cases	14
5 Step-by-Step Guide on How to Get Started with the Intermittent 16/8 Fasting	17
Step 1: Choose Your Eating Window	17
Step 2: Begin Gradually	19
Step 3: Stay Hydrated	22
Step 4: Plan Balanced Meals	24
Step 5: Listen to Your Body	27
Recommended Foods for Intermittent 16/8 Fasting	30
Foods to Avoid	32
General Tips for Avoiding Unhealthy Foods	35
7-Day Sample Meal Plan	36
Easing into the 16-Hour Diet Plan from Days 1 to 5	39
First Set – No Breakfast	39
Second Set – No Dinner	40
Fighting Off Hunger from Days 6 to 10	42
1. Drink lots of fluid.	42
2. Perform work-related tasks.	43
3. Meditate.	44
Staying Motivated from Days 11 to 15	46
Sample Recipes	51
Grilled Chicken Salad	52
Baked Salmon with Quinoa and Steamed Broccoli	53

Turkey and Avocado Wrap	55
Stir-fried tofu with Vegetables and Brown Rice	56
Quinoa and Black Bean Bowl	58
Chicken and Vegetable Skewers	59
Shrimp and Avocado Salad	61
Beef and Veggie Stir-Fry	63
Chickpea and Spinach Curry	66
Baked Chicken Thighs with Sweet Potatoes	68
Tuna Salad Stuffed Peppers	70
Egg and Avocado Toast	72
Zucchini Noodles with Pesto and Chicken	74
Conclusion	**78**
FAQs	**81**
Resources and Helpful Links	**84**

Introduction

If you are looking for an effective fitness strategy that could give you a healthy, trim body, then look no further because you have found the ultimate beginner's guide to the 16-Hour Diet Plan.

This guide contains a step-by-step guide that will show you how to be successful at 16:8 Intermittent Fasting—a type of sporadic diet that requires you to fast for 16 hours and limit your eating times to 8 hours per day. Sounds simple enough, right?

For many people, however, the act of skipping certain meals of the day is not an easy feat to achieve. Various factors in the modern world tend to keep people away from their pursuit of a longer and healthier life.

Therefore, this guide aims to eliminate the popular misconception that effective diet plans are too complicated to understand and follow through. Each chapter of this guide covers the important things that a novice at 16:8 Intermittent Fasting needs to know to successfully adapt to this kind of lifestyle.

In this Guide, you will discover...

- What the 16-Hour Diet is, as well as its advantages over other fitness strategies;
- The numerous health benefits and drawbacks that you should keep in mind before starting this diet plan;
- The ideal meal plan and recipes that you can follow while practicing the 16:8 Intermittent Fasting;
- How to figure out the best fasting and eating schedules that fit with your current lifestyle;
- How to effectively fight off hunger during your fasting periods; and
- How to stay motivated as you continue to engage in intermittent fasting.

This guidebook sets itself apart from the rest through its careful but honest account of what it would take beginners to survive through and complete the 16-Hour Diet Plan. Furthermore, it is also designed for individuals who are seeking to:

- Lose excess body weight
- Improve their existing health condition
- Feel better about themselves

Fasting requires discipline and commitment, but as this guide will show you, it would not demand you to change the way you live your life just so you can attain your personal health goals.

Keep reading and learn more about the 16:8 Intermittent Fasting, and how it can positively impact your life. From understanding the basics of this diet plan to creating a sustainable eating schedule, this guide will equip you with all the necessary information to successfully practice intermittent fasting. Get ready to embark on a journey towards a healthier and happier lifestyle!

What Is Intermittent 16/8 Fasting?

Intermittent 16/8 fasting is a widely adopted eating pattern characterized by fasting for 16 hours and limiting your eating to an 8-hour window each day. This approach differs significantly from traditional diets, which typically concentrate on the types of food you consume.

Instead, 16/8 fasting focuses on timing, creating a cycle that encourages your body to utilize its stored fat for energy during the fasting periods. This method not only aids in weight loss but also improves metabolic health, making it a popular choice for those looking to enhance their overall well-being without strictly monitoring their food intake.

Principles of the Intermittent 16/8 Fasting Method

The 16/8 fasting method is based on the principle of giving your body a longer period without food to promote fat burning, followed by an eating window to nourish and refuel your body. Here are some key principles of this approach:

1. ***Fasting Period***: This period lasts for 16 hours, starting after your last meal and ending with the first meal of your eating window.
2. ***Eating Window***: During this 8-hour time frame, you can consume all of your daily calories and nutrients.
3. ***Consistency***: The success of intermittent fasting depends on consistency. It's essential to maintain a regular schedule and stick to it as closely as possible.
4. ***Proper Nutrition***: While there are no strict guidelines for what you can eat during your eating window, it's crucial to nourish your body with healthy, whole foods to reap the full benefits of this method.

By following these principles, you can effectively implement the 16/8 fasting method into your lifestyle and see positive results.

Benefits of the Intermittent 16/8 Fasting Method

Incorporating the 16/8 fasting method into your lifestyle can offer numerous health benefits, including:

1. ***Weight Loss***: By restricting the time frame for eating, intermittent fasting can help reduce daily calorie intake and promote fat burning, leading to weight loss.
2. ***Better Insulin Sensitivity***: As insulin levels drop during fasting periods, our bodies become more sensitive to insulin, helping regulate blood sugar levels

and potentially preventing conditions like type 2 diabetes.
3. ***Improved Heart Health***: Some studies suggest that intermittent fasting can improve heart health by reducing cholesterol levels and blood pressure.
4. ***Increased Energy***: Many people report feeling more energized during their fasting state as the body switches to using stored fat for energy instead of relying on food.
5. ***Simplified Meal Planning***: With only an 8-hour eating window, meal planning and preparation can become easier and more efficient, leading to potential time and money savings.

When implementing the 16/8 fasting method, it's crucial to listen to your body and adjust accordingly. It's essential to maintain a balanced diet and ensure you're getting enough nutrients during your eating window.

Disadvantages

When done correctly, intermittent fasting can be a beneficial tool for overall health and weight management. However, it's essential to mention some potential disadvantages of the 16/8 method, including:

1. ***Initial Hunger and Cravings***: When starting out, many people experience hunger pangs and cravings

during the fasting window. This can make it challenging to stick to the routine initially.
2. **Social Inconvenience**: Social gatherings and meals with family or friends might not always align with your eating window, making it difficult to adhere to the schedule without feeling left out.
3. **Possible Nutrient Deficiency**: If not carefully planned, intermittent fasting can lead to nutrient deficiencies. Skipping meals may result in missing out on essential vitamins and minerals if the diet isn't well-balanced during the eating window.
4. **Overeating Risk**: Some individuals might overeat or choose unhealthy foods during the eating window, which can negate the benefits of fasting and potentially lead to weight gain or other health issues.
5. **Impact on Fitness Performance**: For some, exercising in a fast state may lead to reduced performance or energy levels. It might take time to find the optimal timing for workouts within the fasting framework.
6. **Digestive Issues**: Rapidly consuming large meals after a fasting period can sometimes cause digestive discomfort, such as bloating or indigestion.

Although there are potential disadvantages to implementing intermittent fasting, the benefits often outweigh them. With proper planning and listening to your body, intermittent fasting can lead to significant time and money savings.

How Does the Intermittent 16/8 Fasting Work?

Intermittent 16/8 fasting works by tapping into our body's natural processes and promoting fat burning. When we eat, our bodies release insulin to help regulate blood sugar levels and store excess calories as fat for later use. During fasting periods, insulin levels drop, allowing our bodies to access stored fat for energy instead of relying on food intake.

Additionally, intermittent fasting has been shown to activate autophagy—a process in which damaged cells are broken down and recycled within the body. This cellular clean-up helps improve overall health and may have anti-aging benefits.

Use Cases

Intermittent 16/8 fasting is utilized for various health and lifestyle benefits. Here are some of the primary use cases:

1. *Type 2 Diabetes*: Intermittent fasting can improve insulin sensitivity and lower blood sugar levels, making it beneficial for managing type 2 diabetes.

2. ***Obesity***: By promoting weight loss and reducing body fat, 16/8 fasting can help manage obesity and reduce its associated health risks.
3. ***Cardiovascular Diseases***: Fasting can improve heart health by lowering cholesterol levels, reducing blood pressure, and decreasing inflammation, which helps manage cardiovascular diseases.
4. ***Metabolic Syndrome***: Improvements in insulin sensitivity, reduced inflammation, and weight loss associated with intermittent fasting can aid in managing metabolic syndrome, which is a cluster of conditions increasing the risk of heart disease, stroke, and diabetes.
5. ***Non-Alcoholic Fatty Liver Disease (NAFLD)***: Weight loss and improved metabolic health from intermittent fasting can reduce liver fat and improve liver function, aiding in the management of NAFLD.
6. ***Hypertension (High Blood Pressure)***: By helping to reduce body weight and improve cardiovascular health, intermittent fasting can contribute to lowering high blood pressure.
7. ***Inflammatory Conditions***: Intermittent fasting has been shown to reduce markers of inflammation in the body, which can help manage chronic inflammatory conditions such as rheumatoid arthritis and other inflammatory diseases.

8. *Alzheimer's Disease*: Some studies suggest that intermittent fasting may support brain health and reduce the risk of neurodegenerative diseases like Alzheimer's by promoting autophagy (cellular repair) and reducing oxidative stress.
9. *Polycystic Ovary Syndrome (PCOS)*: Intermittent fasting may help manage PCOS by improving insulin sensitivity, supporting weight loss, and balancing hormones.
10. *Gastrointestinal Disorders*: Conditions like irritable bowel syndrome (IBS) might be managed better through structured eating times, potentially leading to improved digestive health and symptom control.

While intermittent 16/8 fasting offers potential benefits for managing these diseases, individual responses can vary, and it's important to consult with a healthcare provider before starting any new dietary regimen, especially if you have existing health conditions.

5 Step-by-Step Guide on How to Get Started with the Intermittent 16/8 Fasting

Incorporating intermittent fasting into your lifestyle can be a bit daunting at first, especially if you are new to it. However, with proper guidance and preparation, the 16/8 intermittent fasting can become an easy and sustainable weight loss strategy for you. Here's a step-by-step guide on how to get started:

Step 1: Choose Your Eating Window

Selecting the right 8-hour eating window is crucial for maintaining consistency and fitting into your daily routine. The goal is to find a time frame that aligns with your natural eating habits and lifestyle, making it easier to adhere to the fasting schedule long-term. Here are some common options and their benefits:

- *12 PM to 8 PM*: This window suits those who prefer to skip breakfast and enjoy a late dinner. By starting your eating period at noon, you can have a substantial lunch, an afternoon snack, and a fulfilling dinner. This schedule is great for individuals who may have busy mornings or prefer to extend their social activities into the evening.

- *10 AM to 6 PM*: Ideal for those who like to start their day with a meal and have an earlier dinner. This option allows you to have breakfast, lunch, and an early dinner, which can be beneficial if you need to go to bed early or avoid late-night eating. It's also suitable for people who have a structured workday ending in the early evening.
- *1 PM to 9 PM*: Perfect for night owls who tend to be more active and social in the evenings. This window allows for a later lunch, an afternoon snack, and a late dinner. It accommodates those who might have evening engagements and prefer to eat dinner later in the day.

Tips for Choosing Your Window

1. ***Consider your work schedule***: Align your eating window with your busiest times of the day. For instance, if your mornings are packed with meetings or tasks, opting for a later start time might prevent distractions from hunger.
2. ***Social life and family commitments***: If you often have social dinners or family meals, choose a window that allows you to participate without feeling left out.

Consistency is key, so select a period that you can stick to even on weekends and special occasions.
3. ***Natural hunger patterns***: Pay attention to when you naturally feel hungry. If you're not typically hungry in the morning, skipping breakfast might be easy. Conversely, if you wake up hungry, an earlier window could be more sustainable.
4. ***Daily routine***: Stick to the same window daily to establish a routine. Consistency helps regulate your body's internal clock, making fasting easier over time. Regularity can also improve digestion and optimize energy levels throughout the day.

By carefully considering these factors, you can choose an 8-hour eating window that feels natural and manageable, setting yourself up for success with the 16/8 fasting method. This thoughtful approach will help ensure that intermittent fasting becomes a sustainable part of your lifestyle rather than a short-lived experiment.

Step 2: Begin Gradually

Jumping straight into a 16-hour fast can be challenging, especially if you're not used to extended periods without food. A gradual approach helps your body and mind adjust more comfortably, making it easier to maintain the fasting regimen long-term. Here's how to ease into the 16/8 fasting method:

1. ***Start with a 12-hour fast***: Begin by fasting for 12 hours each day. For instance, stop eating at 8 PM and have your first meal at 8 AM the next day. This 12-hour window often aligns naturally with sleep patterns and is a manageable starting point for most people. It allows your body to get used to fasting overnight while still having ample time to eat during the day.
2. ***Extend to 14 hours***: After a few days or a week of fasting for 12 hours, extend your fasting window by two hours. For example, stop eating at 8 PM and break your fast at 10 AM. This incremental increase helps your body adapt to a slightly longer fasting period without causing significant discomfort.
3. ***Reach 16 hours***: Finally, progress to the full 16-hour fast by stopping eating at 8 PM and having your first meal at 12 PM the following day. This step completes the transition to the 16/8 fasting method, where you'll be fasting for 16 hours and eating within an 8-hour window.

Tips for Transitioning

1. ***Make small adjustments daily or weekly***: Don't rush the process. Gradually increasing your fasting window by 15-30 minutes each day or every few days can make the transition smoother. Small, consistent

changes are less likely to cause hunger pangs or energy dips, making it easier to stick to the plan.
2. ***Stay consistent***: Consistency is key to allowing your body to adapt comfortably. Try to maintain the same fasting schedule every day, even on weekends. Regularity helps regulate your body's internal clock, improves metabolic efficiency, and reduces hunger signals during fasting periods.
3. ***Listen to your body***: Pay attention to how your body responds during the transition. If you experience severe hunger, dizziness, or fatigue, consider slowing down the progression. It's important to strike a balance between challenging yourself and ensuring your well-being.
4. ***Stay hydrated***: Drinking plenty of water during your fasting period can help manage hunger and maintain energy levels. Hydration supports overall health and can make the fasting experience more comfortable.
5. ***Plan your meals***: Knowing what and when you'll eat can help you stick to the fasting schedule. Plan balanced, nutrient-dense meals to ensure you're getting the necessary nutrients within your eating window, which can also help curb cravings during your fasting period.

By taking a gradual approach and listening to your body's cues, you'll be more likely to successfully adopt and maintain the 16/8 fasting method. This measured transition ensures that intermittent fasting becomes a sustainable part of your lifestyle rather than a short-lived experiment.

Step 3: Stay Hydrated

Hydration is a crucial aspect of successful intermittent fasting, particularly during your fasting periods. Drinking plenty of fluids helps reduce hunger pangs, maintain energy levels, and support overall health. Here's an in-depth look at how to stay hydrated and the types of beverages that can be consumed without breaking your fast:

Acceptable Beverages During Fasting

- *Water*: Aim to drink at least 8 glasses (64 ounces) of water each day. Water is essential for maintaining bodily functions, aiding digestion, and keeping you feeling full. Staying well-hydrated can help suppress unnecessary hunger signals and prevent dehydration, which can sometimes be mistaken for hunger.
- *Black Coffee*: Consuming black coffee in moderation can boost metabolism and curb appetite without adding any calories. Coffee contains caffeine, which can increase alertness and energy levels during your fasting period. Just be sure not to add sugar, milk, or cream, as these can break your fast.
- *Herbal Tea*: Herbal teas offer hydration and can be soothing. Many herbal teas, such as peppermint, chamomile, or ginger tea, have additional benefits like

aiding digestion or reducing stress. Since they contain no calories, they won't break your fast and can be enjoyed throughout the day.
- *Sparkling Water*: Sparkling water adds variety and can help with satiety due to its fizz. It can be a refreshing alternative to plain water and might make it easier to drink enough fluids. Choose unsweetened versions to avoid any hidden calories or artificial sweeteners.

Tips for Staying Hydrated

1. *Carry a water bottle*: Having a water bottle with you at all times makes it easier to sip throughout the day. Opt for a reusable bottle, which is environmentally friendly and can help you track your water intake.
2. *Start your day with a large glass of water*: Begin each morning by drinking a large glass of water. This habit kickstarts your hydration for the day and can also help wake up your digestive system.
3. *Set reminders*: If you often forget to drink water, set reminders on your phone or use a hydration-tracking app. These tools can prompt you to take sips regularly and ensure you meet your daily water intake goals.
4. *Flavor your water*: If you find plain water boring, try infusing it with slices of fresh fruit, cucumber, or herbs like mint. Infused water can be more enjoyable to drink and still provides the necessary hydration without added sugars or calories.

5. ***Avoid sugary drinks and sodas***: Even during your eating windows, steer clear of sugary beverages and sodas. These drinks can lead to blood sugar spikes and crashes, undermining the benefits of intermittent fasting. Instead, focus on consuming whole foods and nutrient-dense drinks that support your overall health.
6. ***Monitor your body's signals***: Pay attention to signs of dehydration such as dry mouth, headache, dizziness, or dark urine. If you notice any of these symptoms, increase your fluid intake promptly.

By prioritizing hydration and choosing the right beverages, you can enhance your fasting experience, reduce feelings of hunger, and maintain stable energy levels. Proper hydration supports your body's functions and contributes significantly to the success of your 16/8 fasting regimen.

Step 4: Plan Balanced Meals

Within your eating window, it's crucial to focus on nutrient-dense foods that provide essential nutrients and support overall health. Eating balanced meals helps you feel satiated, maintains energy levels, and maximizes the benefits of intermittent fasting. Here's an expanded look at what to include in your diet and tips for effective meal planning:

Key Nutrients to Include

- ***Protein***: Incorporate a variety of protein sources such as lean meats (chicken, turkey), fish (salmon, tuna),

eggs, beans, legumes (lentils, chickpeas), tofu, and dairy products (Greek yogurt, cottage cheese). Protein is vital for muscle repair and growth, and it also helps keep you full longer. Aim to include a source of protein in every meal to stabilize blood sugar levels and reduce cravings.
- *Healthy Fats*: Healthy fats are essential for brain health, hormone production, and providing lasting energy. Include sources like avocados, nuts (almonds, walnuts), seeds (chia, flax), and oils (olive oil, coconut oil). Fat also adds flavor to meals and can help with the absorption of fat-soluble vitamins (A, D, E, and K).
- *Complex Carbohydrates*: Opt for whole grains (brown rice, quinoa, oats), starchy vegetables (sweet potatoes, butternut squash), and legumes for sustained energy and fiber. Complex carbs are broken down more slowly than simple carbs, providing a steady release of energy and helping maintain stable blood sugar levels.
- *Vegetables and Fruits*: Aim for a variety of colorful produce to ensure you get a wide range of vitamins, minerals, antioxidants, and fiber. Dark leafy greens (spinach, kale), cruciferous vegetables (broccoli, cauliflower), berries, citrus fruits, and other vibrant options contribute to overall health and can help prevent nutrient deficiencies.

Meal Planning Tips

1. ***Prepare your meals ahead of time***: Planning and prepping your meals in advance can help you avoid unhealthy choices when you're hungry. Consider batch cooking on weekends or preparing ingredients in advance (chopping vegetables, marinating proteins) to make weekday meals quicker and easier.
2. ***Include a mix of macronutrients in each meal***: Balance each meal with protein, healthy fats, and complex carbohydrates to keep you full and satisfied longer. For example, a balanced lunch could be grilled chicken (protein) with a quinoa salad (complex carbs) and avocado (healthy fat).
3. ***Avoid processed foods and limit sugar intake***: Processed foods often have added sugars, unhealthy fats, and artificial ingredients that can negate fasting benefits. Focus on whole, minimally processed foods to nourish your body. Limit sugary snacks, desserts, and drinks to maintain stable energy and overall health.
4. ***Stay mindful of portion sizes***: While it's important to eat nutrient-dense foods, be mindful of portion sizes to avoid overeating. Intermittent fasting is not a license to binge eat during your eating window. Listen to your body's hunger and fullness cues to guide your intake.
5. ***Experiment with new recipes***: Keep your meals interesting by trying new recipes and incorporating

different ingredients. This variety not only makes your meals more enjoyable but also ensures you get a diverse range of nutrients.
6. ***Hydrate during your eating window***: Continue to drink water and stay hydrated while eating. Proper hydration supports digestion and helps you feel fuller.

By focusing on balanced, nutrient-rich meals and planning ahead, you can optimize your intermittent fasting experience, enhance overall health, and sustain energy levels throughout the day. Thoughtful meal planning ensures that you're nourishing your body adequately within your eating window and making the most of the 16/8 fasting method.

Step 5: Listen to Your Body

Understanding and responding to your body's signals is crucial for long-term success with intermittent fasting. By tuning into how your body feels and reacts, you can make informed decisions that support your health and well-being. Here's a detailed look at how to listen to your body and tips for monitoring your experience:

Key Considerations

- ***Monitor Hunger Levels***: Pay close attention to your hunger cues. If you find yourself feeling extremely hungry or fatigued, this might indicate that your current fasting window isn't working well for you. You can adjust your eating window or incorporate small, healthy snacks such as a handful of nuts or a piece of fruit during your eating period to help manage hunger. It's important to avoid reaching a point where you're overly hungry, as this can lead to overeating or making unhealthy food choices.

- *Assess Your Energy and Mood*: Track your energy levels and mood throughout the day. Intermittent fasting should leave you feeling energized and balanced. If you experience low energy, irritability, or mood swings, adjust your fasting schedule or evaluate your diet. Ensure you get enough nutrients for your daily activities.
- *Consult a Healthcare Provider*: Before starting any new fasting regimen, especially if you have underlying health conditions such as diabetes, heart disease, or are pregnant, consult with a healthcare provider. A doctor can help tailor a fasting plan that meets your individual health needs and ensure that it's safe for you to proceed.

Tips for Monitoring Your Body

1. *Keep a Journal*: Document your fasting experience by keeping a journal. Note your energy levels, mood, hunger cues, and any physical changes you observe. This record can help you identify patterns and make necessary adjustments. For example, you might notice that you feel more energetic on days when you eat

more protein or when your meals are spaced differently.
2. ***Be Patient***: It takes time for your body to adjust to a new eating pattern. Initial discomfort or changes in energy levels are common as your body adapts to intermittent fasting. Give yourself time to acclimate, and don't be discouraged by early challenges. Patience and consistency are key to seeing the long-term benefits of fasting.
3. ***Make Adjustments as Needed***: Based on your observations and how you feel, don't hesitate to make adjustments. If a 16-hour fast feels too long, try reducing it slightly and gradually work back up. If fasting feels easy, experiment with extending your fasting window. The goal is to find a balance that works for you without causing stress or discomfort.
4. ***Stay Informed and Flexible***: Keep learning about intermittent fasting and nutrition to make informed decisions. Flexibility is important; what works for someone else may not work for you. Tailor the fasting approach to fit your body's unique needs and responses.
5. ***Listen to Cravings***: Sometimes cravings can provide insight into nutritional deficiencies. If you consistently crave certain foods, it might be worth evaluating your diet to ensure you're receiving all necessary nutrients.

For instance, craving sweets might indicate a need for more complex carbohydrates or fiber.

By taking these steps and carefully tuning into your body's signals, you can effectively navigate the intermittent fasting journey. This mindful approach ensures that intermittent fasting becomes a sustainable and beneficial part of your lifestyle, leading to improved health and well-being.

Recommended Foods for Intermittent 16/8 Fasting

When following the 16/8 intermittent fasting method, it's essential to focus on nutrient-dense foods that will provide the energy and nutrients your body needs. Here are some recommended food choices:

Proteins

- *Lean Meats*: Chicken breast, turkey, lean cuts of beef, pork tenderloin
- *Fish and Seafood*: Salmon, tuna, mackerel, shrimp, and other fatty fish rich in omega-3 fatty acids
- *Eggs*: Whole eggs and egg whites
- *Plant-Based Proteins*: Lentils, chickpeas, beans, tofu, tempeh, edamame

Healthy Fats

- *Avocado*: Rich in monounsaturated fats and fiber

- *Nuts and Seeds*: Almonds, walnuts, chia seeds, flaxseeds, pumpkin seeds
- *Oils*: Olive oil, coconut oil, avocado oil
- *Nut Butter*: Peanut butter, almond butter (without added sugars or hydrogenated fats)

Complex Carbohydrates

- *Whole Grains*: Quinoa, brown rice, oatmeal, barley, farro, whole wheat bread, and pasta
- *Vegetables*: Broccoli, spinach, kale, carrots, bell peppers, zucchini, cauliflower, sweet potatoes, Brussels sprouts
- *Fruits*: Berries (strawberries, blueberries, raspberries), apples, oranges, bananas, pears, grapes

Dairy or Dairy Alternatives

- *Dairy*: Greek yogurt, cottage cheese, milk, cheese (in moderation)
- *Dairy Alternatives*: Almond milk, soy milk, oat milk, coconut yogurt

Legumes

- *Beans*: Black beans, kidney beans, pinto beans, navy beans
- *Lentils*: Green, red, brown lentils

Hydration

- *Water*: Essential for staying hydrated throughout both your fasting and eating windows
- *Herbal Teas*: Chamomile, peppermint, and other non-caffeinated teas
- *Black Coffee*: Can help curb appetite during the fasting period (without added sugar or cream)
- *Infused Water*: Water infused with slices of cucumber, lemon, lime, or mint for a refreshing taste

Snacks

- *Fresh Vegetables*: Carrot sticks, celery, cucumber slices, cherry tomatoes
- *Fruits*: Apple slices, berries, grapes
- *Hummus*: Paired with vegetable sticks or whole-grain crackers
- *Greek Yogurt*: With a sprinkle of nuts or seeds

Foods to Avoid

When following the 16/8 intermittent fasting method, it's important to avoid foods that can hinder your progress or negatively impact your health. Here are some foods to avoid:

Sugary Foods

- *Sweets*: Cookies, cakes, candies, pastries.
- *Sugary Drinks*: Sodas, energy drinks, fruit juices with added sugars.

- *Processed Desserts*: Ice cream, chocolate bars, and other high-sugar treats.

Refined Carbohydrates

- *White Bread and Pasta*: Opt for whole-grain versions instead.
- *White Rice*: Choose brown rice or other whole grains.
- *Packaged Snacks*: Crackers, chips, pretzels, and other refined snacks.

Processed Foods

- *Fast Food*: Burgers, fries, fried chicken, and other high-calorie options.
- *Packaged Meals*: Microwave dinners, instant ramen, and other highly processed convenience foods.
- *Processed Meats*: Sausages, hot dogs, bacon, and deli meats with added preservatives and sodium.

Trans Fats and Unhealthy Oils

- *Hydrogenated Oils*: Often found in margarine, shortening, and some processed foods.
- *Fried Foods*: French fries, fried chicken, and other deep-fried items.
- *Commercial Baked Goods*: Store-bought muffins, donuts, and pastries often contain trans fats.

High-Sodium Foods

- *Canned Soups and Processed Meats*: Often contain high levels of sodium and preservatives.
- *Salty Snacks*: Pretzels, salted nuts, and other high-sodium snacks.
- *Restaurant Foods*: Many restaurant dishes, especially from fast food chains, are high in sodium.

Alcohol

- *Beverages*: Beer, wine, cocktails, and other alcoholic drinks can add empty calories and disrupt your fasting schedule.
- *Mixed Drinks*: Cocktails with sugary mixers contribute additional unnecessary calories.

Artificial Ingredients

- *Artificial Sweeteners*: Found in diet sodas, sugar-free candies, and some low-calorie processed foods.
- *Preservatives and Additives*: Common in many processed and packaged foods.

Low-Quality Dairy Products

- *Flavored Yogurts*: Often contain added sugars.
- *Processed Cheese*: Includes cheese slices and cheese spreads containing additives and preservatives.

General Tips for Avoiding Unhealthy Foods

1. **Read Labels**

    Check ingredient lists and nutrition labels to avoid hidden sugars, unhealthy fats, and excessive sodium.

2. **Cook at Home**

    Preparing meals at home allows you to control the ingredients and avoid unhealthy additives.

3. **Avoid Ultra-Processed Foods**

    Stick to whole, minimally processed foods to ensure you're consuming the most nutrients.

By avoiding these foods, you'll better support your health goals and maximize the benefits of the 16/8 intermittent fasting method. Focus on whole, nutrient-dense foods to keep your body fueled and satisfied.

7-Day Sample Meal Plan

To help you kick things off the right way, here is a sample 7-day meal plan that you could follow while easing yourself into your new routine brought about by the 16-Hour Meal Plan.

Since you would be putting your body and mind to a challenge during your fasting periods, you should make it a point to replenish your energy with healthy but nutritious meals as much as possible. In between each meal, you may also consider snacking on nuts and any fruit of your choice.

Here's a sample seven-day meal plan for the 16/8 intermittent fasting method. The eating window is from 12 PM to 8 PM each day. Ensure that your meals are nutritious and balanced, focusing on whole, unprocessed foods.

Day 1

Lunch (12 PM): Grilled Chicken Salad

Snack (3 PM): Mixed Nuts and Berries

Dinner (8 PM): Baked Salmon with Quinoa and Steamed Broccoli

Day 2

Lunch (12 PM): Turkey and Avocado Wrap

Snack (3 PM): Greek Yogurt with Honey and Nuts

Dinner (8 PM): Stir-fried tofu with Vegetables

Day 3

Lunch (12 PM): Quinoa and Black Bean Bowl

Snack (3 PM): Apple Slices with Almond Butter

Dinner (8 PM): Chicken and Vegetable Skewer

Day 4

Lunch (12 PM): Shrimp and Avocado Salad

Snack (3 PM): Carrot Sticks with Hummus

Dinner (8 PM): Beef and Veggie Stir-Fry

Day 5

Lunch (12 PM): Chickpea and Spinach Curry

Snack (3 PM): Cheese and Crackers

Dinner (8 PM): Baked Chicken Thighs with Sweet Potatoes

Lunch (12 PM): Lentil Soup

Snack (3 PM): Hard-Boiled Eggs

Dinner (8 PM): Tuna Salad Stuffed Peppers

Day 7

Lunch (12 PM): Egg and Avocado Toast

Snack (3 PM): Smoothie

Dinner (8 PM): Zucchini Noodles with Pesto and Chicken

This meal plan provides a variety of nutritious and satisfying meals that fit into the 16/8 intermittent fasting schedule. Adjust portion sizes and ingredients as needed to meet your individual dietary needs and preferences.

Easing into the 16-Hour Diet Plan from Days 1 to 5

During the first five days, your goal is to gradually familiarize your body and mind with fasting. Along the way, aim to find the best fasting schedule for your lifestyle.

Some people think starting with a full 16-hour fast is best to reach their goal faster. However, for sustainability and optimal results, start with a 12-hour fast on your first day. Add 1 hour of fasting each day to reach the standard 16 hours.

Here are two suggested fasting and eating cycles for Day 1 to Day 5. The first set leads to skipping breakfast, while the second set means skipping supper by Day 5 and onwards.

First Set – No Breakfast

Day 1

- Duration of Fasting Period: 12 hours
- Suggested Eating Period: from 10 am to 10 pm (12 hours)

Day 2

- Duration of Fasting Period: 13 hours
- Suggested Eating Period: from 11 am to 10 pm (11 hours)

Day 3

- Duration of Fasting Period: 14 hours
- Suggested Eating Period: from 12 noon to 10 pm (10 hours)

Day 4

- Duration of Fasting Period: 15 hours
- Suggested Eating Period: from 12 noon to 9 pm (9 hours)

Day 5

- Duration of Fasting Period: 16 hours
- Suggested Eating Period: from 12 noon to 8 pm (8 hours)

Second Set – No Dinner

Day 1

- Duration of Fasting Period: 12 hours
- Suggested Eating Period: from 9 am to 9 pm (12 hours)

Day 2

- Duration of Fasting Period: 13 hours
- Suggested Eating Period: from 9 am to 8 pm (11 hours)

Day 3

- Duration of Fasting Period: 14 hours
- Suggested Eating Period: from 9 am to 7 pm (10 hours)

Day 4

- Duration of Fasting Period: 15 hours
- Suggested Eating Period: from 9 am to 6 pm (9 hours)

Day 5

- Duration of Fasting Period: 16 hours
- Suggested Eating Period: from 9 am to 5 pm (8 hours)

If you would notice, both the recommended fasting periods cover the normal sleeping hours. They count as fasting hours in the 16-Hour Diet Plan, thus making this weight-loss strategy much easier to manage than you might have initially thought.

Fighting Off Hunger from Days 6 to 10

Now that you've mastered your intermittent fasting schedule, your next goal is to stave off hunger. For Days 6 to 10, you will strictly limit yourself to the standard 8-hour eating period, likely experiencing more frequent and intense hunger pangs during the 16 hours of fasting.

Hunger is a natural sensation, but your reaction to it determines your success. The 16-hour Diet Plan requires discipline, which, like muscle, can be trained to resist hunger. By controlling your reaction, you can avoid cravings and stick to your goals.

Sitting around all day makes resisting hunger harder. Your mind focuses on your bodily sensations. To clear this phase of your fasting journey, here are 5 strategies to stay productive and keep hunger at bay.

1. **Drink lots of fluid.**

    Many fitness experts consider this as the healthiest and simplest method of fighting off hunger during a fast.

Studies show that people usually confuse hunger with thirst. This means that when you feel hungry, your body might actually be craving hydration rather than food. As such, they tend to reach for something to eat rather than something to drink.

Since the 16:8 Intermittent Fasting forbids you from eating anything for 16 hours a day, you would be better off drinking fluids such as water, sparkling water, black coffee, or black tea throughout the day. Carry a water container with you so that you can take sips whenever you feel hungry. Staying hydrated not only helps manage hunger but also keeps your energy levels up and supports overall bodily functions. Including fluids with electrolytes can further help maintain balance, especially during prolonged fasting periods.

2. Perform work-related tasks.

Work is usually a prime source of activities that could keep your mind occupied for long periods. Moreover, the busier you are, the faster the time seems to pass. Therefore, to make your fasting hours more productive and your hunger more manageable, try to focus on finishing your presentation for an important meeting, responding to work emails, or whatever tasks at work that need your attention.

Engaging deeply in work can serve as a powerful distraction from hunger. By immersing yourself in these activities, you not only make the fasting period more bearable but also boost your productivity. Setting specific goals for your workday and breaking down tasks into manageable chunks can help keep your focus sharp and your mind off food.

3. Meditate.

Though meditation isn't essential to fully suppress hunger, it's a powerful tool to better control your thoughts during a fast. For best results, try quick, frequent meditations throughout the day. Beginners should aim for 2 to 4 sessions daily, at 10 minutes each. Use these times to accept hunger as a natural experience and learn to control your reactions to it.

In addition to helping manage hunger, meditation can reduce stress, improve mental clarity, and enhance emotional well-being. Practicing mindfulness during fasting periods allows you to become more attuned to your body's signals and helps cultivate a sense of peace and patience. Consider using guided meditation apps or videos if you're new to the practice, and gradually increase the duration as you become more comfortable.

Don't let hunger stop you from achieving your fitness goals. The hunger you feel during fasting is not the same as true starvation. It's your body's way of adjusting to a new eating pattern. You can manage daily hunger pangs without suffering or overexerting yourself by staying hydrated, keeping busy with productive tasks, and practicing mindfulness. Remember, fasting is a journey that can lead to both physical and mental benefits, so approach it with a positive and patient mindset.

Staying Motivated from Days 11 to 15

When you reach Days 11 to 14 of your journey, you will likely feel the monotony of the 16-Hour Diet Plan. After all, you have just gone through the same cycle for several days at this point.

Consistent eating times and fasting periods, however, are important in unlocking the numerous health benefits of the 16:8 Intermittent Fasting. As such, it is best to stick with the schedule that has worked for you since Day 5.

Fortunately, various techniques could be effective in getting you to stay motivated in your pursuit of a healthier lifestyle. Below are some of the best ones that you should consider practicing yourself.

1. **List down the positive effects of intermittent fasting that you experienced recently.**

    Because you are in the midst of things, you might not be able to notice the progress you have made so far. If that is the case, then consider taking the time to observe the good things that have happened to you as a result of taking on the 16-Hour Diet Plan. Reflect on the changes in your body, your energy levels, and your overall well-being. Think about the days when you felt more energetic, more focused, or simply happier.

Rather than focusing on the things you have not accomplished yet, check out how much weight you have lost since Day 1, or how well you have been eating or sleeping these past few days. Celebrate the small victories, such as fitting into an old pair of jeans, receiving compliments from friends, or simply feeling more comfortable in your own skin. These achievements, no matter how minor they may seem, are important milestones in your journey.

To keep better track of your progress, note down these things in a journal or a blog so that you can look back at these positive changes in your life whenever you are feeling demotivated or frustrated. Write about your experiences, your challenges, and your triumphs. Documenting your journey not only helps you stay motivated but also serves as a valuable resource for others who might be embarking on a similar path. Remember, every step forward, no matter how small, is a step towards a healthier and happier you.

2. **Visualize your ultimate health goals.**

    Picture in your mind how your life would be if you would stick to the 16-Hour Diet Plan. Do not just focus on the images, but also on the feelings and sensations that you could associate with your ideal future. By doing so, you would be able to strengthen the mental pathways that are essential in achieving your goals.

    Visualization exercises are so simple that you can do it in 5 to 10 minutes. If you are not sure how to go about it, just follow these steps:

- Close your eyes, and take slow, deep breaths.
- Think about an incredibly positive and detailed scene related to your goals for doing the 16-Hour Diet Plan.
- Imagine how the scene would play out right from the very start.
- Picture the exact moment you realize that you have attained success.

    If negative thoughts start to creep up on you while doing this, pause for a while to wipe away your doubts and insecurities. Then, restart your efforts by concentrating only on the positive outcomes of your diet plan.

3. **Recite positive affirmations to yourself.**

    Think about positive affirmations that highlight your strengths as a person, the importance of what you are doing, the progress you have made so far, and the ideal future that you want for yourself. These affirmations serve as powerful reminders of your capabilities and the goals you are striving towards. By focusing on these positive thoughts, you can bolster your confidence and motivation.

List them down somewhere accessible to you so that you can recite them to yourself whenever you need a motivational boost. This could be in a journal, on sticky notes around your house, or even as a note on your phone. Having them readily available ensures that you can turn to them in moments of doubt or when you need a quick pick-me-up.

Below are some examples of great positive affirmations for those pursuing the 16:8 Intermittent Fasting:

- I am compassionate, patient, and strong.
- My health is my number one priority.
- I am taking a step each day towards a long and happy life.
- I feel grateful for my good health for allowing me to spend more time with my family and friends.

These affirmations not only reinforce your commitment to intermittent fasting but also remind you of the broader benefits of your efforts, such as improved health and more quality time with loved ones.

You are not required to just choose one at a time though. Figuring out the right combination of motivational tactics for you could significantly increase your chances of successfully adhering to the 16-Hour Diet Plan.

Sample Recipes

Below are some sample recipes to help you get started with your 16-Hour Diet Plan. These are all simple yet nutritious meals that can be prepared in less than an hour, and would make great options for your eating window:

Grilled Chicken Salad

Ingredients:

- 2 boneless, skinless chicken breasts
- Salt and pepper to taste
- 1 tablespoon olive oil
- 6 cups of mixed greens or your choice of lettuce
- 1 medium-sized cucumber, sliced
- 1 cup cherry tomatoes, halved

Instructions:

1. Preheat your grill to medium-high heat.
2. Season the chicken breasts with salt and pepper on both sides.
3. Grill the chicken for about six minutes on each side until fully cooked.
4. Set aside and let it rest for five minutes before slicing into bite-sized pieces.
5. In a separate bowl, mix the lettuce, cucumber, and cherry tomatoes together.
6. Add in the grilled chicken slices on top.
7. You can also add in your choice of dressing.
8. Serve and enjoy!

Baked Salmon with Quinoa and Steamed Broccoli

Ingredients:

- 2 salmon fillets
- Salt and pepper to taste
- 1 tablespoon olive oil
- 1 cup quinoa, rinsed
- 2 cups water or chicken broth for added flavor
- 2 cups broccoli florets

Instructions:

1. Preheat your oven to 375°F.
2. Place the salmon fillets on a baking sheet lined with parchment paper.
3. Season both sides of the salmon with salt and pepper.
4. Drizzle olive oil over the top of the salmon.
5. Bake in the oven for about 12 minutes or until fully cooked.
6. In a separate pot, bring the water or chicken broth to a boil.
7. Add in the quinoa and let it simmer for 15 minutes or until fully cooked.

8. In another pot, steam the broccoli florets for about five minutes.
9. Serve the salmon on top of a bed of quinoa with steamed broccoli on the side.
10. Enjoy this nutritious and filling meal!

Turkey and Avocado Wrap

Ingredients:

- 1 large tortilla wrap
- 4 slices of deli turkey
- 1/2 avocado, mashed
- 1/4 cup shredded cheese

Instructions:

1. Lay the tortilla wrap flat on a clean surface.
2. Spread the mashed avocado evenly over the entire wrap.
3. Place the slices of turkey on top of the mashed avocado.
4. Sprinkle shredded cheese over the turkey.
5. Roll up tightly and cut into smaller pieces if desired.
6. This wrap can be enjoyed as is or heated up in a pan until the cheese melts.
7. Pack it for an easy and satisfying lunch!

Stir-fried tofu with Vegetables and Brown Rice

Ingredients:

- 1 block of extra firm tofu, drained and cubed
- 1 tablespoon sesame oil
- 1 red bell pepper, sliced
- 1 cup broccoli florets
- Salt and pepper to taste
- 2 cups cooked brown rice

Instructions:

1. In a wok or large pan, heat sesame oil over medium-high heat.
2. Add in the cubed tofu and cook until lightly browned on all sides.
3. Remove tofu from the pan and set aside.
4. In the same pan, add in the sliced red bell pepper and broccoli florets.
5. Cook for about 5 minutes or until vegetables are tender.
6. Season with salt and pepper to taste.

7. Add the cooked tofu back into the pan and stir to combine with the vegetables.
8. Serve over a bed of brown rice and enjoy this protein-packed plant-based meal!
9. Feel free to add any other veggies or sauces of your choice for added flavor and variety.

Quinoa and Black Bean Bowl

Ingredients:

- 1 cup quinoa
- 2 cups water or vegetable broth
- 1 can black beans, drained and rinsed
- 1 red bell pepper, diced
- 1 avocado, diced
- Fresh cilantro for garnish (optional)

Instructions:

1. In a pot, bring the quinoa and water/broth to a boil.
2. Lower heat to a simmer and cover for about 15 minutes.
3. Fluff with a fork and let cool for a few minutes.
4. In a separate pan, sauté the bell pepper until slightly soft.
5. Add in the black beans and cook until heated through.
6. In a bowl, mix together the cooked quinoa, black bean and bell pepper mixture, and diced avocado.
7. Garnish with fresh cilantro if desired.

This nutrient-dense bowl is a great option for a quick and healthy lunch. Feel free to add in any other vegetables or protein of your choice to make it even more satisfying.

Chicken and Vegetable Skewers

Ingredients:

- 1 pound chicken breast, cut into cubes
- 2 tablespoons olive oil
- 2 cloves garlic, minced
- 1 teaspoon dried oregano
- Salt and pepper to taste
- Assorted vegetables of your choice (such as bell peppers, onions, mushrooms)

Instructions:

1. In a bowl, mix together the olive oil, minced garlic, oregano, salt and pepper.
2. Add in the cubed chicken and marinate for at least 30 minutes or up to overnight in the fridge.
3. Preheat the grill to medium-high heat.
4. Assemble skewers by alternating pieces of marinated chicken with vegetables.
5. Grill skewers for about 10 minutes on each side, or until chicken is fully cooked and vegetables are slightly charred.
6. Serve with a side of rice or quinoa for a complete meal.

This grilled dish is perfect for summer gatherings or as a quick weeknight dinner option. You can also switch up the marinade by using different herbs and spices to add variety to your meals.

Shrimp and Avocado Salad

Ingredients:

For the Shrimp:

- 1 lb large shrimp, peeled and deveined
- 1 tablespoon olive oil
- 2 cloves garlic, minced
- 1 teaspoon smoked paprika
- Salt and pepper to taste

For the Salad:

- 4 cups mixed greens (spinach, arugula, or romaine lettuce)
- 1 avocado, diced
- 1 cup cherry tomatoes, halved
- 1 cucumber, sliced
- 1/4 red onion, thinly sliced
- 1/4 cup fresh cilantro, chopped

For the Dressing:

- 3 tablespoons olive oil
- 2 tablespoons lime juice
- 1 teaspoon honey or maple syrup
- 1 teaspoon Dijon mustard
- Salt and pepper to taste

Instructions:

1. Combine the olive oil, minced garlic, smoked paprika, salt, and pepper in a large bowl, mixing thoroughly.
2. Add in the cleaned shrimp and toss to coat evenly.
3. Let marinate for at least 15 minutes or up to an hour in the fridge.
4. Preheat the grill to medium-high heat.
5. Grill shrimp for about 3-4 minutes on each side, until pink and cooked through.
6. In a separate bowl, whisk together all the ingredients for the dressing until well combined.
7. In a large salad bowl, combine mixed greens, avocado, cherry tomatoes, cucumber, red onion, and cilantro.
8. Add in grilled shrimp and drizzle with dressing before serving.

This refreshing salad is packed with nutrients and healthy fats from the avocado and shrimp. It's a great dish to add to your meal rotation for a light and flavorful option. You can also serve it as an appetizer or side dish at any summer barbecue or cookout.

Beef and Veggie Stir-Fry

Ingredients:

For the Beef Marinade:

- 1 lb beef sirloin or flank steak, thinly sliced
- 2 tablespoons low-sodium soy sauce or tamari (for gluten-free)
- 1 tablespoon olive oil or sesame oil
- 1 tablespoon rice vinegar
- 2 cloves garlic, minced
- 1 teaspoon freshly grated ginger
- 1 teaspoon honey or maple syrup (optional)

For the Stir-Fry:

- 1 red bell pepper, sliced into strips
- 1 yellow bell pepper, sliced into strips
- 1 cup broccoli florets
- 1 carrot, julienned
- 1 cup snap peas, trimmed
- 1/2 cup sliced mushrooms
- 2 green onions, sliced
- 2 tablespoons low-sodium soy sauce or tamari
- 1 tablespoon olive oil or sesame oil
- 1 clove garlic, minced
- 1 teaspoon freshly grated ginger

For Serving:

- Cooked brown rice or cauliflower rice
- Sesame seeds (optional)
- Fresh cilantro, chopped (optional)

Instructions:

1. Combine beef slices with soy sauce or tamari, olive oil or sesame oil, rice vinegar, minced garlic, grated ginger, and honey or maple syrup (optional). Let marinate for at least 30 minutes in the fridge.
2. In the meantime, prepare your veggies by slicing the bell peppers into thin strips, julienning the carrot, trimming snap peas, and slicing mushrooms. Set aside.
3. Heat a wok or large skillet over medium-high heat with 1 tablespoon of olive oil or sesame oil.
4. Add in marinated beef slices and cook until browned on both sides (about 5-6 minutes). Transfer to a plate and set aside.
5. In the same pan, add sliced bell peppers, broccoli florets, julienned carrot, snap peas, and sliced mushrooms. Cook for about 3-4 minutes until veggies are slightly softened.
6. Add green onions, minced garlic, and grated ginger to the pan. Stir-fry for another 2 minutes.

7. Return cooked beef slices to the pan with the veggies. Pour in soy sauce or tamari and stir-fry for an additional 1-2 minutes until everything is well coated.
8. Serve your beef stir-fry over cooked brown rice or cauliflower rice. Top with sesame seeds and chopped cilantro (optional).
9. Enjoy your delicious and nutritious beef stir-fry!

Chickpea and Spinach Curry

Ingredients:

For the Curry:

- 1 tablespoon olive oil or coconut oil
- 1 large onion, finely chopped
- 3 cloves garlic, minced
- 1 tablespoon freshly grated ginger
- 1 teaspoon ground cumin
- 1 teaspoon ground coriander
- 1 teaspoon turmeric powder
- 1/2 teaspoon ground cinnamon
- 1/2 teaspoon smoked paprika
- 1/4 teaspoon cayenne pepper (optional, for heat)
- 1 can (15 oz) diced tomatoes
- 1 can (15 oz) coconut milk (full-fat or light, depending on preference)
- 1 can (15 oz) chickpeas, drained and rinsed
- 4 cups fresh spinach, roughly chopped
- Salt and pepper to taste

For Serving:

- Cooked brown rice, quinoa, or cauliflower rice
- Fresh cilantro, chopped (optional)
- Lime wedges (optional)

Instructions:

1. Heat olive oil or coconut oil in a large skillet or saucepan over medium heat.
2. Add chopped onion, minced garlic, and grated ginger to the pan. Cook for about 3-4 minutes until onions are translucent.
3. Stir in ground cumin, coriander, turmeric powder, cinnamon, smoked paprika, and cayenne pepper (if using). Cook for an additional 1-2 minutes until fragrant.
4. Pour in diced tomatoes with their juices and stir well.
5. Add a can of coconut milk and drained chickpeas to the pan. Bring to a gentle boil then reduce heat to low and let simmer for about 10 minutes.
6. Stir in roughly chopped spinach to the curry and let it wilt down for a couple of minutes.
7. Season with salt and pepper to taste.
8. Serve the curry over cooked brown rice, quinoa, or cauliflower rice.
9. Optional: Garnish with freshly chopped cilantro and squeeze some lime juice over the top for added flavor.

Baked Chicken Thighs with Sweet Potatoes

Ingredients:

For the Chicken:

- 6 bone-in, skin-on chicken thighs
- 2 tablespoons olive oil
- 2 cloves garlic, minced
- 1 teaspoon dried rosemary
- 1 teaspoon dried thyme
- 1 teaspoon smoked paprika
- Salt and pepper to taste
- Juice of 1 lemon

For the Sweet Potatoes:

- 2 large sweet potatoes, peeled and cut into 1-inch cubes
- 1 tablespoon olive oil
- 1 teaspoon ground cinnamon
- 1/2 teaspoon smoked paprika
- Salt and pepper to taste

For Garnish (Optional):

- Fresh parsley, chopped
- Lemon wedges

Instructions:

1. Preheat your oven to 375°F (190°C). Grease a large baking dish with olive oil.
2. In a small bowl, mix together the minced garlic, dried rosemary, thyme, smoked paprika, salt, pepper, and lemon juice.
3. Use your hands to rub the spice mixture onto both sides of the chicken thighs.
4. Place the chicken thighs in the prepared baking dish and set aside.
5. In a separate bowl, toss together the sweet potato cubes with olive oil, ground cinnamon, smoked paprika, salt, and pepper until evenly coated.
6. Arrange the sweet potatoes around the chicken thighs in the baking dish.
7. Bake for 35-40 minutes or until chicken is fully cooked and reaches an internal temperature of 165°F (74°C).
8. Serve the chicken and sweet potatoes together on a platter.
9. Optional: Garnish with chopped parsley and serve with lemon wedges for added flavor.

Tuna Salad Stuffed Peppers

Ingredients:

For the Tuna Salad:

- 2 cans (5 oz each) tuna packed in water, drained
- 1/4 cup Greek yogurt (or mayonnaise if preferred)
- 1 tablespoon Dijon mustard
- 1 celery stalk, finely chopped
- 1 small red onion, finely chopped
- 1 small cucumber, finely chopped
- 1 tablespoon fresh dill, chopped (optional)
- Juice of 1 lemon
- Salt and pepper to taste

For the Peppers:

- 4 large bell peppers (red, yellow, or orange), halved and seeds removed

For Garnish (Optional):

- Fresh parsley, chopped

Instructions:

1. Preheat your oven to 375°F (190°C). Place the halved peppers in a large baking dish.
2. In a medium bowl, mix together the canned tuna, Greek yogurt (or mayonnaise), Dijon mustard, celery, red onion, cucumber, and dill (if using).

3. Squeeze lemon juice over the mixture and season with salt and pepper to taste.
4. Spoon the tuna salad into each pepper half until all are filled.
5. Bake for 20-25 minutes or until the peppers are tender and the filling is heated through.
6. Serve the stuffed peppers on a platter and garnish with chopped parsley if desired.

Egg and Avocado Toast

Ingredients:

For the Toast:

- 2 slices whole grain or sourdough bread
- 1 ripe avocado
- 1 tablespoon lemon juice
- Salt and pepper to taste

For the Eggs:

- 2 large eggs
- 1 teaspoon olive oil or butter
- Salt and pepper to taste

For Garnish (Optional):

- Red pepper flakes
- Fresh cilantro or parsley, chopped
- Cherry tomatoes, halved

Instructions:

1. Toast the bread slices until golden brown.
2. In a small bowl, mash the avocado with lemon juice, salt, and pepper to create a spread.
3. Heat a medium-sized skillet over medium heat and add olive oil or butter.

4. Crack each egg into the skillet and cook for about 2-3 minutes on each side until the desired level of doneness is reached.
5. Spread the mashed avocado onto each toast slice and top with a cooked egg.
6. Garnish with red pepper flakes, fresh herbs, or cherry tomatoes if desired.
7. Serve immediately for a delicious and nutrient-packed breakfast or snack!

Zucchini Noodles with Pesto and Chicken

Ingredients:

For the Chicken:

- 2 boneless, skinless chicken breasts
- 1 tablespoon olive oil
- Salt and pepper to taste
- 1 teaspoon Italian seasoning

For the Zucchini Noodles:

- 4 medium zucchinis, spiralized into noodles (zoodles)
- 1 tablespoon olive oil
- 2 cloves garlic, minced
- Salt and pepper to taste

For the Pesto:

- 2 cups fresh basil leaves
- 1/4 cup pine nuts or walnuts
- 1/2 cup grated Parmesan cheese
- 2 cloves garlic
- 1/2 cup olive oil
- Salt and pepper to taste
- Juice of 1 lemon (optional, for extra freshness)

For Garnish (Optional):

- Cherry tomatoes, halved
- Fresh basil leaves

- Extra grated Parmesan cheese

Instructions:

1. Preheat oven to 375°F.
2. In a small bowl, mix together olive oil, salt, pepper, and Italian seasoning.
3. Place chicken breasts in a baking dish and brush the olive oil mixture on both sides of the chicken.
4. Bake for 25-30 minutes, or until the chicken is fully cooked.
5. While the chicken is cooking, make the zucchini noodles by spiralizing the zucchini into noodles using a vegetable spiralizer.
6. Heat a large skillet over medium heat and add olive oil and minced garlic.
7. Add the zucchini noodles to the skillet and season with salt and pepper to taste.
8. Cook for about 2-3 minutes until softened but still slightly crunchy.
9. To make the pesto, combine basil leaves, pine nuts or walnuts, Parmesan cheese, garlic, and olive oil in a food processor or blender.
10. Blend until smooth and creamy.
11. Once the chicken is fully cooked, remove it from the oven and let it rest for 5 minutes before slicing it into strips.

12. In a large mixing bowl, toss the zucchini noodles with the pesto sauce until well coated.
13. Serve the zucchini noodles on plates or bowls and top with sliced chicken strips.
14. Garnish with halved cherry tomatoes, fresh basil leaves, and extra-grated Parmesan cheese if desired.

Incorporating diverse, nutritious meals into your 16/8 intermittent fasting plan can enhance both enjoyment and health benefits. The provided recipes ensure a balanced intake of proteins, healthy fats, and essential nutrients, supporting sustained energy and overall well-being.

These meals fit dietary restrictions while offering flavorful options to keep you satisfied and nourished. By focusing on high-quality ingredients and mindful preparation, you can maximize the benefits of intermittent fasting, making it a sustainable and enjoyable approach to a healthy lifestyle.

Conclusion

Thank you for reading this guide on Intermittent 16/8 fasting. You've started a journey with the potential to improve your health and well-being. By finishing this guide, you've shown commendable commitment and curiosity, essential for any lifestyle change.

Remember, intermittent fasting isn't just a diet; it's a sustainable lifestyle choice. You've learned the basics of the 16/8 method, its benefits, and how to integrate it into your daily routine. Whether you aim to lose weight, improve metabolic health, or adopt a healthier eating pattern, the 16/8 method offers a flexible framework.

One of the most promising aspects of intermittent fasting is its array of health benefits. From increased energy levels to improved mental clarity, the positive changes you'll notice can be both immediate and long-lasting. By restricting your eating window, you're giving your body the time it needs to repair and rejuvenate, which can lead to better overall health.

Implementing the 16/8 fasting method can be straightforward, especially with the right tips and strategies. Start by choosing an eating window that suits your lifestyle. For many, a window from 12 PM to 8 PM works well, but feel free to adjust it according to your personal schedule. Consistency is key, so try to stick to the same hours every day.

Stay hydrated throughout your fasting period. Drinking water, herbal teas, or black coffee can help curb hunger and keep you energized. When it's time to eat, focus on nutrient-dense foods that provide essential vitamins and minerals. Balanced meals with a good mix of protein, healthy fats, and complex carbohydrates will keep you satisfied and nourished.

Like any lifestyle change, intermittent fasting has its challenges. You might feel initial hunger pangs or struggle to adapt to a new eating schedule, but these usually subside as your body adjusts. Be patient and remember your reasons for starting. Keeping a food journal or connecting with others practicing intermittent fasting can offer support and motivation.

Intermittent fasting is a personal journey, so listen to your body. What works for one person might not work for another, so adjust the method to fit your needs. Celebrate your progress, no matter how small, and don't be too hard on yourself if you face setbacks. Every step towards a healthier lifestyle is progress.

Remember, the goal is not perfection but progress. By committing to the 16/8 fasting method, you're making a conscious decision to prioritize your health. This decision alone is a significant achievement and should be celebrated.

As you continue your intermittent fasting journey, remember that the benefits go beyond physical health. The discipline and mindfulness needed for fasting can positively impact other areas of your life. You'll likely become more aware of your eating habits and more intentional in your choices, leading to a balanced and fulfilling lifestyle.

Thank you for reading this guide. Your dedication to improving your health is inspiring. Stay curious, committed, and kind to yourself. Here's to your success on the path to a healthier, happier you!

If you need a refresher or additional tips, feel free to revisit this guide. Your journey is ongoing, and every resource you use brings you closer to your goals. Happy fasting!

FAQs

What is the 16/8 fasting method?

The 16/8 fasting method involves fasting for 16 hours and eating all your meals within an 8-hour window. For example, you might eat between 12 PM and 8 PM and fast from 8 PM to 12 PM the next day. This pattern helps your body to cycle between periods of eating and fasting.

Can I drink liquids during the fasting period?

Yes, you can drink non-caloric beverages like water, herbal teas, and black coffee during the fasting period. These drinks can help keep you hydrated and may even help curb hunger pangs. Just be sure to avoid adding any sugar, cream, or other additives that contain calories.

Will intermittent fasting help me lose weight?

Many people find that intermittent fasting helps them lose weight by reducing their overall calorie intake and improving metabolic health. By limiting your eating window, you may naturally consume fewer calories without the need for strict calorie counting. Additionally, fasting can help improve insulin sensitivity and promote fat burning.

Is 16/8 fasting safe for everyone?

While 16/8 fasting is generally safe for most healthy adults, it may not be suitable for everyone. Pregnant or breastfeeding women, individuals with a history of eating disorders, and those with certain medical conditions should consult their healthcare provider before starting any fasting regimen. It's essential to listen to your body and prioritize your health.

Can I exercise while fasting?

Yes, you can exercise while fasting, but it's important to pay attention to how your body responds. Some people find they have more energy and better performance when working out in a fast state, while others may need to adjust their workout intensity. Start with lighter exercises and gradually increase intensity as you become more accustomed to fasting.

What should I eat during my eating window?

Focus on nutrient-dense, whole foods that provide essential vitamins and minerals. Include a balance of lean proteins, healthy fats, and complex carbohydrates in your meals. Examples of healthy foods to include are vegetables, fruits, whole grains, lean meats, fish, nuts, and seeds. Avoid processed foods, sugary snacks, and excessive amounts of refined carbohydrates.

How long does it take to see results with 16/8 fasting?

The time it takes to see results can vary depending on individual factors such as starting weight, diet, and activity level. Some people may notice changes in energy levels and appetite control within a few days, while others might take a few weeks to see significant weight loss or other health benefits. Consistency is key, so stick with the 16/8 method and give your body time to adapt.

Resources and Helpful Links

Leonard, J. (2023b, October 2). A guide to 16:8 intermittent fasting. https://www.medicalnewstoday.com/articles/327398#:~:text=It%20involves%20fasting%20for%2016,and%20other%20obesity%2Dassociated%20conditions.

Ld, L. S. M. R. (2023c, August 1). What is 16/8 intermittent fasting? A beginner's guide. Healthline. https://www.healthline.com/nutrition/16-8-intermittent-fasting

BSc, K. G. (2024, May 3). Intermittent Fasting 101 — The Ultimate Beginner's guide. Healthline. https://www.healthline.com/nutrition/intermittent-fasting-guide

Vetter, C. (2024, April 18). Intermittent fasting: What can you eat or drink? https://zoe.com/learn/what-to-eat-or-drink-while-intermittent-fasting

Intermittent Fasting: What is it, and how does it work? (2023, September 29). Johns Hopkins Medicine. https://www.hopkinsmedicine.org/health/wellness-and-prevention/intermittent-fasting-what-is-it-and-how-does-it-work

Stanton, B. (2023, May 11). 16/8 Intermittent Fasting: A Beginner's Guide. Carb Manager. https://www.carbmanager.com/article/zdaoqraaajeomvdd/168-intermittent-fasting-a-beginners-guide

Kieszkowska, K. (2023, April 3). Intermittent fasting. Naturally Balanced. https://naturallybalanced.org/en/intermittent-fasting/

Lange, M., Nadkarni, D., Martin, L., Newberry, C., Kumar, S., & Kushner, T. (2023). Intermittent fasting improves hepatic end points in nonalcoholic fatty liver disease: A systematic review and meta-analysis. Hepatology Communications, 7(8). https://doi.org/10.1097/hc9.0000000000000212

www.ingramcontent.com/pod-product-compliance
Lightning Source LLC
LaVergne TN
LVHW010428070526
838199LV00066B/5961

For many people, however, the act of skipping certain meals of the day is not an easy feat to achieve. Various factors in the modern world tend to keep people away from their pursuit of a longer and healthier life.

Therefore, this guide aims to eliminate the popular misconception that effective diet plans are too complicated to understand and follow through. Each chapter of this book covers the important things that a novice at 16:8 Intermittent Fasting needs to know in order to successfully adapt to this kind of lifestyle.

With these points in mind, you will discover…
- What the 16-Hour Diet is, as well as its advantages over other fitness strategies;
- The numerous health benefits and drawbacks that you should keep in mind before starting this diet plan;
- The ideal meal plan and recipes that you can follow while practicing the 16:8 Intermittent Fasting;
- How to figure out the best fasting and eating schedules that fit with your current lifestyle;
- How to effectively fight off hunger during your fasting periods; and
- How to stay motivated as you continue to engage in intermittent fasting.
-

This guide sets itself apart from the rest through its careful but honest account of what it would take for beginners to survive through and successfully complete the 16-Hour Diet Plan.

Occipital Neuralgia

A BEGINNER'S GUIDE AND OVERVIEW TO MANAGING THE CONDITION THROUGH DIET, WITH SAMPLE CURATED RECIPES

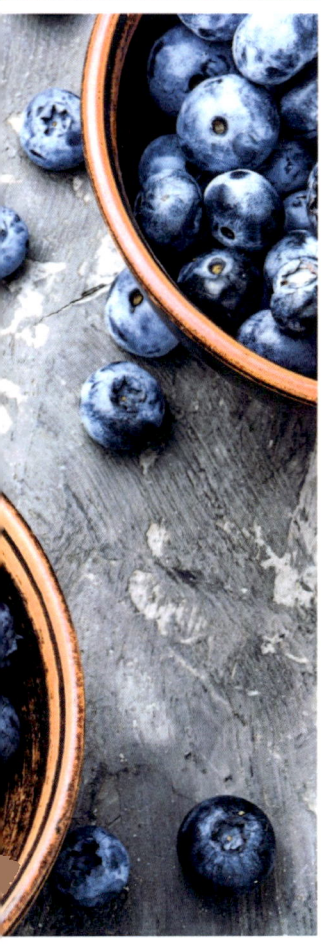
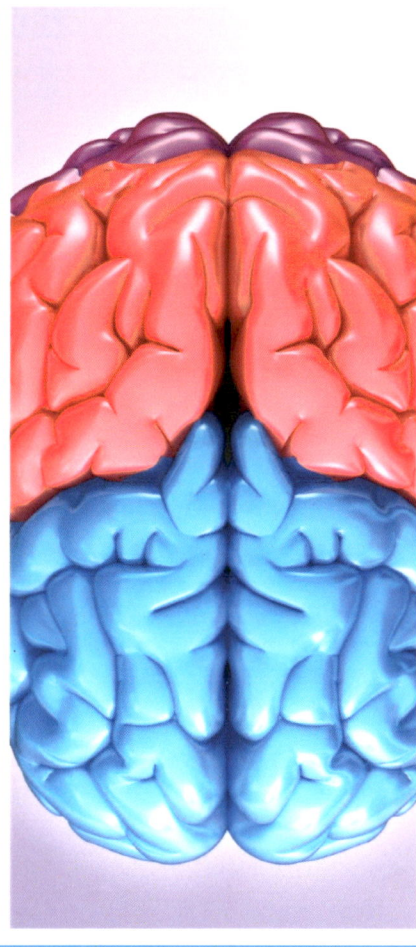
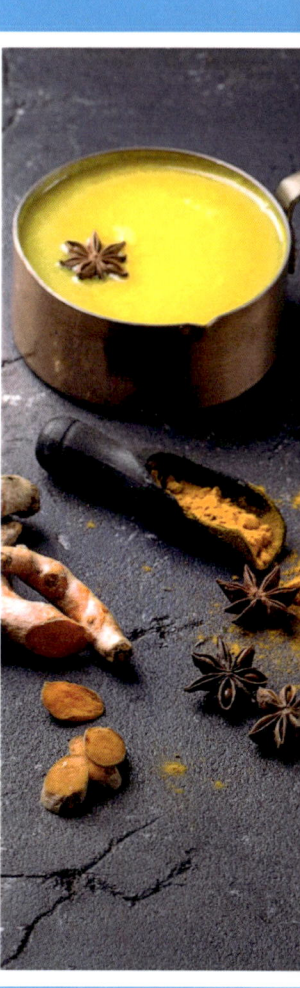

Patrick Marshwell